REGIONAL ITALIAN RECIPES 2021

DELICIOUS RECIPES TO MAKE AT HOME

SECOND EDITION

MEAT, VEGETABLES AND PASTRIES

ز

MIKE SANTORO

BUON

APPETITO!!!

TABLE OF CONTENTS

Roast Leg of Lamb with Potatoes, Garlic, and Rosemary

Agnello al Forno

Makes 6 servings

Italians would serve this lamb well done, but I think it tastes best when medium-rare, which is about 130°F on an instant-read thermometer. Let the lamb rest after roasting it so that the juices have a chance to retreat to the center of the meat.

6 all-purpose potatoes, peeled and cut into 1-inch chunks

3 tablespoons olive oil

Salt and freshly ground black pepper

1 bone-in leg of lamb, trimmed (about 5½ pounds)

6 garlic cloves, finely chopped

2 tablespoons chopped fresh rosemary

1. Place a rack in the middle of the oven. Preheat oven to 350°F. Place the potatoes in a roasting pan large enough to hold the meat and potatoes without crowding. Toss with the oil, and salt and pepper to taste.

2. Make shallow slits all over the lamb with a small knife. Poke some of the garlic and rosemary into the slits, reserving a little for the potatoes. Sprinkle the meat generously with salt and pepper. Push the potatoes aside and add the meat fat-side up.

3. Place the pan in the oven and cook 30 minutes. Turn the potatoes. Roast 30 to 45 minutes longer or until the internal temperature measures 130°F on an instant-read thermometer placed in the thickest part of the meat, away from the bone. Remove the pan from the oven and transfer the lamb to a cutting board. Cover the meat with foil. Let rest at least 15 minutes before slicing.

4. Test the potatoes for doneness by piercing them with a sharp knife. If they need further cooking, turn the oven up to 400°F., return the pan to the oven, and cook until tender.

5. Slice the lamb and serve hot with the potatoes.

Leg of Lamb with Lemon, Herbs, and Garlic

Agnello Steccato

Makes 6 servings

Basil, mint, garlic, and lemon perfume this lamb roast. Once it is in the oven, there is not much else to do. It is the perfect dish for a small dinner party or a Sunday dinner. Add some potatoes, carrots, turnips, or other root vegetables to the roasting pan, if you like.

1 shank-end leg of lamb, well trimmed (about 3 pounds)

2 garlic cloves

2 tablespoons chopped fresh basil

1 tablespoon chopped fresh mint

¼ cup freshly grated Pecorino Romano or Parmigiano-Reggiano

1 teaspoon grated lemon zest

½ teaspoon dried oregano

Salt and freshly ground black pepper

2 tablespoons olive oil

1. Place a rack in the center of the oven. Preheat the oven to 425°F.

2. Very finely chop the garlic, basil, and mint. In a small bowl, stir the mixture together with the cheese, lemon zest, and oregano. Stir in 1 teaspoon salt and freshly ground pepper to taste. With a small knife, make slits about $3/4$-inch deep all over the meat. Stuff a little of the herb mixture into each slit. Rub the oil all over the meat. Roast for 15 minutes.

3. Turn the heat down to 350°F. Roast 1 hour more or until the meat is medium-rare and the internal temperature reaches 130°F on an instant-read thermometer placed in the thickest part but not touching the bone.

4. Remove the lamb from the oven and transfer to a cutting board. Cover the lamb with foil and let rest 15 minutes before carving. Serve hot.

Braised Lamb–Stuffed Zucchini

Zucchine Ripiene

Makes 6 servings

A leg of lamb feeds a crowd, but after a small dinner party, I often have leftovers. That's when I make these tasty stuffed zucchini. Other types of cooked meat or even poultry can be substituted.

2 to 3 (½-inch thick) slices Italian bread

¼ cup milk

1 pound cooked lamb

2 large eggs

2 tablespoons chopped fresh flat-leaf parsley

2 garlic cloves, finely chopped

½ cup freshly grated Pecorino Romano or Parmigiano-Reggiano

Salt and freshly ground black pepper

6 medium zucchini, scrubbed and trimmed

2 cups tomato sauce, such as Marinara Sauce

1. Place a rack in the center of the oven. Preheat the oven to 425°F. Oil a 13 × 9 × 2–inch baking pan.

2. Remove the bread crust and tear the bread into pieces. (You should have about 1 cup.) Place the pieces into a medium bowl, pour on the milk, and let soak.

3. In a food processor, chop the meat very fine. Transfer to a large bowl. Add the eggs, parsley, garlic, soaked bread, $1/4$ cup of the cheese, and salt and pepper to taste. Mix well.

4. Cut the zucchini in half lengthwise. Scoop out the seeds. Stuff the zucchini with the meat mixture. Place the zucchini side by side in the pan. Spoon on the sauce and sprinkle with the remaining cheese.

5. Bake 35 to 40 minutes or until the stuffing is cooked through and the zucchini are tender. Serve hot or at room temperature.

Rabbit with White Wine and Herbs

Coniglio al Vino Bianco

Makes 4 servings

This is a basic rabbit recipe from Liguria that can be varied by adding black or green olives or other herbs. Cooks in this region prepare rabbit in many different ways, including with pine nuts, mushrooms, or artichokes.

1 rabbit (2½ to 3 pounds), cut into 8 pieces

Salt and freshly ground black pepper

3 tablespoons olive oil

1 small onion, finely chopped

½ cup finely chopped carrot

½ cup finely chopped celery

1 tablespoon chopped fresh rosemary leaves

1 teaspoon chopped fresh thyme

1 bay leaf

½ cup dry white wine

1 cup chicken broth

1. Rinse the rabbit pieces and pat dry with paper towels. Sprinkle with salt and pepper.

2. In a large skillet, heat the oil over medium heat. Add the rabbit and brown lightly on all sides, about 15 minutes.

3. Scatter the onion, carrot, celery, and herbs around the rabbit pieces and cook until the onion is softened, about 5 minutes.

4. Add the wine and bring it to a simmer. Cook until most of the liquid is evaporated, about 2 minutes. Add the broth and bring it to a simmer. Reduce the heat to low. Cover the pan and cook, turning the rabbit occasionally with tongs, until tender when pierced with a fork, about 30 minutes.

5. Transfer the rabbit to a serving platter. Cover and keep warm. Increase the heat and boil the contents of the skillet until reduced and syrupy, about 2 minutes. Discard the bay leaf.

6. Pour the contents of the pan over the rabbit and serve immediately.

Rabbit with Olives

Coniglio alla Stimperata

Makes 4 servings

Red pepper, green olives, and capers flavor this Sicilian-style rabbit dish. The term alla stimperata is given to a number of Sicilian recipes, though its meaning is not clear. It may stem from stemperare, meaning "to dissolve, dilute, or mix" and referring to the addition of water to the pot as the rabbit cooks.

1 rabbit (2½ to 3 pounds), cut into 8 pieces

¼ cup olive oil

3 garlic cloves, chopped

1 cup pitted green olives, rinsed and drained

2 red bell peppers, cut into thin strips

1 tablespoon capers, rinsed

Pinch of oregano

Salt and freshly ground black pepper

2 tablespoons white wine vinegar

½ cup water

1. Rinse the rabbit pieces and pat dry with paper towels.

2. In a large skillet, heat the oil over medium heat. Add the rabbit and brown the pieces well on all sides, about 15 minutes. Transfer the rabbit pieces to a plate.

3. Add the garlic to the skillet and cook 1 minute. Add the olives, pepper, capers, and oregano. Cook, stirring 2 minutes.

4. Return the rabbit to the pan. Season with salt and pepper to taste. Add the vinegar and water and bring to a simmer. Reduce the heat to low. Cover and cook, turning the rabbit occasionally, until the rabbit is tender when pierced with a fork, about 30 minutes. Add a little water if the liquid evaporates. Transfer to a serving platter and serve hot.

Rabbit, Porchetta Style

Coniglio in Porchetta

Makes 4 servings

The combination of seasonings used to make roast pork is so delicious that cooks have adapted it to other meats that are more convenient to cook. Wild fennel is used in the Marches region, but dried fennel seed can be substituted.

1 rabbit (2½ to 3 pounds), cut into 8 pieces

Salt and freshly ground black pepper

2 tablespoons olive oil

2 ounces pancetta

3 garlic cloves, finely chopped

2 tablespoons chopped fresh rosemary

1 tablespoon fennel seeds

2 or 3 sage leaves

1 bay leaf

1 cup dry white wine

$\frac{1}{2}$ cup water

1. Rinse the rabbit pieces and pat them dry with paper towels. Sprinkle with salt and pepper.

2. In a skillet large enough to hold the rabbit pieces in a single layer, heat the oil over medium heat. Place the pieces in the pan. Scatter the pancetta all around. Cook until the rabbit is browned on one side, about 8 minutes.

3. Turn the rabbit and scatter the garlic, rosemary, fennel, sage, and bay leaf all around. When the rabbit is browned on the second side, after about 7 minutes, add the wine and stir, scraping the bottom of the pan. Simmer the wine for 1 minute.

4. Cook uncovered, turning the meat occasionally, until the rabbit is very tender and coming away from the bone, about 30 minutes. (Add a little water if the pan becomes too dry.)

5. Discard the bay leaf. Transfer the rabbit to a serving platter and serve hot with the pan juices.

Rabbit with Tomatoes

Coniglio alla Ciociara

Makes 4 servings

In the Ciociara region outside Rome, known for its delicious cooking, rabbit is braised in tomato sauce and white wine.

1 rabbit (2½ to 3 pounds), cut into 8 pieces

2 tablespoons olive oil

2 ounces pancetta, thickly sliced and chopped

2 tablespoons chopped fresh flat-leaf parsley

1 garlic clove, lightly smashed

Salt and freshly ground black pepper

1 cup dry white wine

2 cups peeled, seeded, and chopped plum tomatoes

1. Rinse the rabbit pieces, then pat dry with paper towels. Heat the oil in a large skillet over medium heat. Place the rabbit in the pan, then add the pancetta, parsley, and garlic. Cook until the rabbit is nicely browned on all sides, about 15 minutes. Sprinkle with salt and pepper.

2. Remove the garlic from the pan and discard it. Stir in the wine and simmer 1 minute.

3. Reduce the heat to low. Stir in the tomatoes, then cook until the rabbit is tender and coming away from the bone, about 30 minutes.

4. Transfer the rabbit to a serving platter and serve hot with the sauce.

Sweet-and-Sour Braised Rabbit

Coniglio in Agrodolce

Makes 4 servings

Sicilians are known for their sweet tooth, a legacy of the Arab domination of the island that lasted at least two hundred years. Raisins, sugar, and vinegar give this rabbit a mildly sweet-and-sour flavor.

1 rabbit (2½ to 3 pounds), cut into 8 pieces

2 tablespoons olive oil

2 ounces thickly sliced pancetta, chopped

1 medium onion, finely chopped

Salt and freshly ground black pepper

1 cup dry white wine

2 whole cloves

1 bay leaf

1 cup beef or chicken broth

1 tablespoon sugar

¼ cup white wine vinegar

2 tablespoons raisins

2 tablespoons pine nuts

2 tablespoons chopped fresh flat-leaf parsley

1. Rinse the rabbit pieces, then pat dry with paper towels. In a large skillet, heat the oil and pancetta over medium heat for 5 minutes. Add the rabbit and cook on one side until browned, about 8 minutes. Turn the rabbit pieces with tongs and scatter the onion all around. Sprinkle with salt and pepper.

2. Add the wine, cloves, and bay leaf. Bring the liquid to a simmer and cook until most of the wine has evaporated, about 2 minutes. Add the broth and cover the pan. Reduce the heat to low and cook until the rabbit is tender, 30 to 45 minutes.

3. Transfer the rabbit pieces to a plate. (If there is a lot of liquid left, boil it over high heat until reduced.) Stir in the sugar, vinegar, raisins, and pine nuts. Stir until the sugar dissolves, about 1 minute.

4. Return the rabbit to the pan and cook, turning the pieces in the sauce, until they seem well coated, about 5 minutes. Stir in the parsley and serve hot with the pan juices.

Roasted Rabbit with Potatoes

Coniglio Arrosto

Makes 4 servings

At my friend Dora Marzovilla's home, a Sunday dinner or special occasion meal often begins with an assortment of tender, crisp fried vegetables, such as artichoke hearts or asparagus, followed by steaming bowls of homemade orecchiette or cavatelli tossed with a delicious ragù made with tiny meatballs. Dora, who comes from Rutigliano in Puglia, is a wonderful cook, and this rabbit dish, which she serves as the main course, is one of her specialties.

1 rabbit (2½ to 3 pounds), cut into 8 pieces

¼ cup olive oil

1 medium onion, finely chopped

2 tablespoons chopped fresh flat-leaf parsley

½ cup dry with wine

Salt and freshly ground black pepper

4 medium all-purpose potatoes, peeled and cut into 1-inch wedges

½ cup water

½ teaspoon oregano

1. Rinse the rabbit pieces and pat dry with paper towels. In a large skillet, heat two tablespoons of the oil over medium heat. Add the rabbit, onion and parsley. Cook, turning the pieces occasionally, until lightly browned, about 15 minutes. Add the wine and cook 5 minutes more. Sprinkle with salt and pepper.

2. Place a rack in the center of the oven. Preheat the oven to 425°F. Oil a roasting pan large enough to hold all of the ingredients in a single layer.

3. Scatter the potatoes in the pan and toss them with the remaining 2 tablespoons oil. Add the contents of the skillet to the pan, tucking the rabbit pieces around the potatoes. Add the water. Sprinkle with the oregano and salt and pepper. Cover the pan with aluminum foil. Roast 30 minutes. Uncover and cook 20 minutes more or until the potatoes are tender.

4. Transfer to a serving platter. Serve hot.

Marinated Artichokes

Carciofi Marinati

Makes 6 to 8 servings

These artichokes are excellent in salads, with cold cuts, or as part of an antipasto assortment. The artichokes will last at least two weeks in the refrigerator.

If baby artichokes are not available, substitute medium artichokes, cut into eight wedges.

1 cup white wine vinegar

2 cups water

1 bay leaf

1 whole garlic clove

8 to 12 baby artichokes, trimmed and quartered (see To prepare whole artichokes)

Pinch of crushed red pepper

Salt

Extra-virgin olive oil

1. In a large saucepan, combine the vinegar, water, bay leaf, and garlic. Bring the liquid to a simmer.

2. Add the artichokes, crushed red pepper, and salt to taste. Cook until tender when pierced with a knife, 7 to 10 minutes. Remove from the heat. Pour the contents of the pan through a fine-mesh strainer into a bowl. Reserve the liquid.

3. Pack the artichokes into sterilized glass jars. Pour in the cooking liquid to cover. Let cool completely. Cover and refrigerate at least 24 hours or up to 2 weeks.

4. To serve, drain the artichokes and toss them with oil.

Roman-Style Artichokes

Carciofi alla Romana

Makes 8 servings

Small farms all around Rome produce loads of fresh artichokes during the spring and fall artichoke seasons. Little trucks bring them to the street-corner markets, where they are sold right off the back of the truck. The artichokes have long stems and leaves still attached, because the stems, once peeled, are good to eat. Romans cook artichokes with the stem side up. They look very appealing when laid out on a serving platter.

2 large garlic cloves, finely chopped

2 tablespoons chopped fresh flat-leaf parsley

1 tablespoon chopped fresh mint or ½ teaspoon dried marjoram

Salt and freshly ground black pepper

¼ cup olive oil

8 medium artichokes, prepared for stuffing (see To prepare whole artichokes)

½ cup dry white wine

1. In a small bowl, stir together the garlic, parsley, and mint or marjoram. Add salt and pepper to taste. Stir in 1 tablespoon of the oil.

2. Gently spread the leaves of the artichokes and push some of the garlic mixture down into the center. Squeezing the artichokes slightly to hold in the filling, place them stem-side up in a pan just large enough to hold them upright. Pour the wine around the artichokes. Add water to a depth of $3/4$ inch. Drizzle the artichokes with the remaining oil.

3. Cover the pan and bring the liquid to a simmer over medium heat. Cook 45 minutes or until the artichokes are tender when pierced with a knife. Serve hot or at room temperature.

Braised Artichokes

Carciofi Stufati

Makes 8 servings

Artichokes are members of the thistle family, and they grow on low bushy plants. They are found wild in many places in southern Italy, and many people cultivate them in their home gardens. An artichoke is actually an unopened flower. Very large artichokes grow at the top of the bush, while small ones sprout near the base. The small artichokes, often called baby artichokes, are great for braising. Prepare them for cooking as you would a larger artichoke. Their buttery sweet flavor and texture is especially good with fish.

1 small onion, finely chopped

$\frac{1}{4}$ cup olive oil

1 garlic clove, finely chopped

2 tablespoons chopped fresh flat-leaf parsley

2 pounds baby artichokes, trimmed and cut into quarters

$\frac{1}{2}$ cup water

Salt and freshly ground black pepper

1. In a large saucepan, cook the onion in the oil over medium heat until tender, about 10 minutes. Stir in the garlic and parsley.

2. Place the artichokes in the pan and stir well. Add the water and salt and pepper to taste. Cover and cook over low heat until the artichokes are tender when pierced with a knife, about 15 minutes. Serve warm or at room temperature.

Variation: In Step 2, add 3 medium potatoes, peeled and cut into 1-inch cubes, with the onion.

Artichokes, Jewish Style

Carciofi alla Giudia

Makes 4 servings

Jewish people first arrived in Rome in the first century B.C. They
settled near the Tiber River and in 1556 were confined to a walled
ghetto by Pope Paul IV. Many were poor, and they made do with
whatever simple, inexpensive foods were available, such as salt cod,
zucchini, and artichokes. By the time the ghetto walls came down in
the mid-1800s, the Jews of Rome had developed their own style of
cooking, which later became fashionable with other Romans. Today,
Jewish dishes such as fried stuffed zucchini blossoms, Semolina
Gnocchi, and these artichokes are considered Roman classics.

The Jewish Quarter of Rome still exists, and there are several good
restaurants where you can sample this style of cooking. At Piperno
and Da Giggetto, two favorite trattorias, these fried artichokes are
served hot with plenty of salt. The leaves are as crisp as potato chips.
The artichokes spatter as they cook, so stand back from the stove
and protect your hands.

4 medium artichokes, prepared as for stuffing

Olive oil

Salt

1. Pat the artichokes dry. Place an artichoke with the bottom up on a flat surface. With the heel of your hand, press down on the artichoke to flatten it and spread the leaves open. Repeat with the remaining artichokes. Turn them so the leaf tips face up.

2. In a large deep skillet or wide heavy saucepan, heat about 2 inches of the olive oil over medium heat until an artichoke leaf slipped into the oil sizzles and browns quickly. Protect your hand with an oven mitt, as the oil can spit and spatter if the artichokes are moist. Add the artichokes with leaf tips down. Cook, pressing the artichokes down into the oil with a slotted spoon until browned on one side, about 10 minutes. With tongs, carefully turn the artichokes and cook until browned, about 10 minutes more.

3. Drain on paper towels. Sprinkle with salt and serve immediately.

Roman Spring Vegetable Stew

La Vignarola

Makes 4 to 6 servings

Italians are very much in tune with the seasons, and the arrival of the first spring artichokes indicates that winter is over and warm weather will soon be returning. To celebrate, Romans eat bowls of this fresh spring vegetable stew, featuring artichokes, as a main course.

4 ounces sliced pancetta, chopped

¼ cup olive oil

1 medium onion, chopped

4 medium artichokes, trimmed and quartered

1 pound fresh fava beans, shelled, or substitute 1 cup frozen fava or lima beans

$^1/_2$ cup Chicken Broth

Salt and freshly ground black pepper

1 pound fresh peas, shelled (about 1 cup)

2 tablespoons chopped fresh flat-leaf parsley

1. In a large frying pan, cook the pancetta in the oil over medium heat. Stir frequently until the pancetta begins to brown, 5 minutes. Add the onion and cook until golden, about 10 minutes more.

2. Add the artichokes, fava beans, broth, and salt and pepper to taste. Lower the heat. Cover and cook 10 minutes or until the artichokes are almost tender when pierced with a knife. Add the peas and parsley and cook 5 minutes more. Serve hot or at room temperature.

Crispy Artichoke Hearts

Carciofini Fritti

Makes 6 to 8 servings

In the United States, artichokes are grown primarily in California, where they were first planted in the early twentieth century by Italian immigrants. The varieties are different from those in Italy, and they are often very mature when picked, so that they are sometimes tough and woody. Frozen artichoke hearts can be very good and save a lot of time. I sometimes use them for this recipe. Fried artichoke hearts are delicious with lamb chops or as an appetizer.

12 baby artichokes, trimmed and quartered, or 2 (10-ounce) packages frozen artichoke hearts, slightly undercooked according to package directions

3 large eggs, beaten

Salt

2 cups plain dry bread crumbs

Oil for frying

Lemon wedges

1. Pat the fresh or cooked artichokes dry. In a medium shallow bowl, beat the eggs with salt to taste. Spread the bread crumbs on a sheet of wax paper.

2. Place a wire cooling rack over a baking sheet. Dip the artichokes in the egg mixture, then roll them in the crumbs. Place the artichokes on the rack to dry at least 15 minutes before cooking.

3. Line a tray with paper towels. Pour oil to a depth of 1 inch in a large heavy skillet. Heat the oil until a drop of the egg mixture sizzles. Add just enough of the artichokes to fit comfortably in the pan without crowding. Cook, turning the pieces with tongs, until golden brown, about 4 minutes. Drain on the paper towels and keep warm while frying the remaining artichokes, in batches if necessary.

4. Sprinkle with salt and serve hot with the lemon wedges.

Stuffed Artichokes

Carciofi Ripieni

Makes 8 servings

This is the way my mother always made artichokes—it's a classic preparation all over southern Italy. There is only enough stuffing to season the artichokes and enhance their flavor. Too much stuffing gets soggy and makes the artichokes heavy, so don't increase the amount of bread crumbs, and of course use crumbs from good-quality bread. The artichokes can be made ahead of time and served at room temperature or eaten hot and freshly made.

8 medium artichokes, prepared for stuffing

¾ cup plain dry bread crumbs

¼ cup chopped fresh flat-leaf parsley

¼ cup freshly grated Pecorino Romano or Parmigiano-Reggiano

1 garlic clove, very finely chopped

Salt and freshly ground black pepper

Olive oil

1. With a large chef's knife, finely chop the artichoke stems. Mix the stems in a large bowl with the bread crumbs, parsley, cheese, garlic, and salt and pepper to taste. Add a little oil and toss to moisten the crumbs evenly. Taste and adjust the seasoning.

2. Gently spread the leaves apart. Lightly stuff the center of the artichokes with the bread crumb mixture, also adding a little stuffing between the leaves. Do not pack the stuffing in.

3. Stand the artichokes in a pot just wide enough to hold them upright. Add water to a depth of $3/4$ inch around the artichokes. Drizzle the artichokes with 3 tablespoons olive oil.

4. Cover the pot and place it over medium heat. When the water comes to a simmer, reduce the heat to low. Cook about 40 to 50 minutes (depending on the size of the artichokes) or until the artichoke bottoms are tender when pierced with a knife and a leaf pulls out easily. Add additional warm water if needed to prevent scorching. Serve warm or at room temperature.

Sicilian-Style Stuffed Artichokes

Carciofi alla Siciliana

Makes 4 servings

The hot dry climate of Sicily is perfect for growing artichokes. The plants, which have jagged, silvery leaves, are quite beautiful, and many people use them as decorative shrubs in their home gardens. At the end of the season, artichokes left on the plant open all the way, exposing the fully matured choke at the center, which is purple and brushy.

This is the Sicilian way of stuffing artichokes, which is more complex than the Stuffed Artichokes recipe. Serve as a first course before roasted fish or a leg of lamb.

4 medium artichokes, prepared for stuffing

½ cup plain bread crumbs

4 anchovy fillets, finely chopped

2 tablespoons chopped drained capers

2 tablespoons pine nuts, toasted

41

2 tablespoons golden raisins

2 tablespoons chopped fresh flat-leaf parsley

1 large garlic clove, finely chopped

Salt and freshly ground black pepper

4 tablespoons olive oil

$\frac{1}{2}$ cup dry white wine

Water

1. In a medium bowl, combine the bread crumbs, anchovies, capers, pine nuts, raisins, parsley, garlic, and salt and pepper to taste. Stir in two tablespoons of the oil.

2. Gently spread the leaves apart. Stuff the artichokes loosely with the bread crumb mixture, also adding a little stuffing between the leaves. Do not pack the stuffing in.

3. Stand the artichokes in a pot just large enough to hold them upright. Add water to a depth of $3/4$ inch around the artichokes. Drizzle with the remaining 2 tablespoons oil. Pour the wine around the artichokes.

4. Cover the pot and place it over medium heat. When the water comes to a simmer, reduce the heat to low. Cook 40 to 50 minutes (depending on the size of the artichokes) or until the artichoke bottoms are tender when pierced with a knife and a leaf pulls out easily. Add additional warm water if needed to prevent scorching. Serve warm or at room temperature.

Asparagus "In the Pan"

Asparagi in Padella

Makes 4 to 6 servings

These asparagus are quickly stir-fried. Add chopped garlic or fresh herbs, if you like.

3 tablespoons olive oil

1 pound asparagus

Salt and freshly ground black pepper

2 tablespoons chopped fresh flat-leaf parsley

1. Trim off the base of the asparagus at the point where the stem turns from white to green. Cut the asparagus into 2-inch lengths.

2. In a large skillet, heat the oil over medium heat. Add the asparagus and salt and pepper to taste. Cook 5 minutes, stirring often, or until the asparagus are lightly browned.

3. Cover the pan and cook 2 minutes more or until the asparagus are just tender. Stir in the parsley and serve immediately.

Asparagus with Oil and Vinegar

Insalata di Asparagi

Makes 4 to 6 servings

As soon as the first locally grown spears appear in the spring, I prepare them this way and eat a big batch to satisfy the craving that has developed through the long winter. Turn the asparagus in the dressing while they are still warm so that they absorb the flavor.

1 pound asparagus

Salt

¼ cup extra-virgin olive oil

1 to 2 tablespoons red wine vinegar

Freshly ground black pepper

1. Trim off the base of the asparagus at the point where the stem turns from white to green. Bring about 2 inches of water to a boil in a large skillet. Add the asparagus and salt to taste. Cook until the asparagus bend slightly when you lift them from the stem end, 4 to 8 minutes. Cooking time will depend on the thickness of the asparagus. Remove the asparagus with tongs. Drain on paper towels and pat them dry.

2. In a large shallow dish, combine the oil, vinegar, a pinch of salt, and a generous grind of pepper. Whisk with a fork until blended. Add the asparagus and turn them gently until coated. Serve warm or at room temperature.

Asparagus with Lemon Butter

Asparagi al Burro

Makes 4 to 6 servings

Asparagus cooked this basic way goes with practically everything, from eggs to fish to meat. Add chopped fresh chives, parsley, or basil to the butter as a variation.

1 pound asparagus

Salt

2 tablespoons unsalted butter, melted

1 tablespoon fresh lemon juice

Freshly ground black pepper

1. Trim off the base of the asparagus at the point where the stem turns from white to green. Bring about 2 inches of water to a boil in a large skillet. Add the asparagus and salt to taste. Cook until the asparagus bend slightly when you lift them from the stem end, 4 to 8 minutes. Cooking time will depend on the thickness of the asparagus. Remove the asparagus with tongs. Drain them on paper towels and pat them dry.

2. Wipe out the skillet. Add the butter and cook over medium heat until melted, about 1 minute. Stir in the lemon juice. Return the asparagus to the pan. Sprinkle them with pepper and turn them gently to coat with the sauce. Serve immediately.

Asparagus with Various Sauces

Makes 4 to 6 servings

Plain boiled asparagus are wonderful served at room temperature with different sauces. They are great for a dinner party because they can be made ahead. It doesn't matter whether they are thick or thin, but try to get asparagus that are all pretty much the same size, so that they cook evenly.

Olive Oil Mayonnaise, Orange Mayonnaise, or Green Sauce

1 pound asparagus

Salt

1. Prepare the sauce or sauces, if necessary. Then, trim off the base of the asparagus at the point where the stem turns from white to green.

2. Bring about 2 inches of water to a boil in a large skillet. Add the asparagus and salt to taste. Cook until the asparagus bend slightly when you lift them from the stem end, 4 to 8 minutes. Cooking time will depend on the thickness of the asparagus.

3. Remove the asparagus with tongs. Drain them on paper towels and pat them dry. Serve the asparagus at room temperature with one or more of the sauces.

Asparagus with Caper-Egg Dressing

Asparagi con Caperi e Uove

Makes 4 to 6 servings

In Trentino–Alto Adige and the Veneto, thick white asparagus are a rite of spring. They are fried and boiled, added to risottos, soups, and salads. An egg dressing is a typical condiment, such as this one with lemon juice, parsley, and capers.

1 pound asparagus

Salt

¼ cup olive oil

1 teaspoon fresh lemon juice

Freshly ground pepper

1 hard cooked egg, diced

2 tablespoons chopped fresh flat-leaf parsley

1 tablespoon capers, rinsed and drained

1. Trim off the base of the asparagus at the point where the stem turns from white to green. Bring about 2 inches of water to a boil in a large skillet. Add the asparagus and salt to taste. Cook until the asparagus bend slightly when you lift them from the stem end, 4 to 8 minutes. Cooking time will depend on the thickness of the asparagus. Remove the asparagus with tongs. Drain them on paper towels and pat them dry.

2. In a small bowl, whisk together the oil, lemon juice, and a pinch of salt and pepper. Stir in the egg, parsley, and capers.

3. Place the asparagus on a serving platter and spoon on the sauce. Serve immediately.

Asparagus with Parmesan and Butter

Asparagi alla Parmigiana

Makes 4 to 6 servings

This is sometimes called asparagi alla Milanese—asparagus, Milan style—though it is eaten in many different regions. If you can find white asparagus, they take particularly well to this treatment.

1 pound thick asparagus

Salt

2 tablespoons unsalted butter

Freshly ground black pepper

½ cup freshly grated Parmigiano-Reggiano

1. Trim off the base of the asparagus at the point where the stem turns from white to green. Bring about 2 inches of water to a boil in a large skillet. Add the asparagus and salt to taste. Cook until the asparagus bend slightly when you lift them from the stem end, 4 to 8 minutes. Cooking time will depend on the thickness of the asparagus. Remove the asparagus with tongs. Drain them on paper towels and pat them dry.

2. Place a rack in the center of the oven. Preheat the oven to 450°F. Butter a large baking dish.

3. Arrange the asparagus side by side in the baking dish, overlapping them slightly. Dot with butter and sprinkle with pepper and the cheese.

4. Bake 15 minutes or until the cheese is melted and golden. Serve immediately.

Asparagus and Prosciutto Bundles

Fagottini di Asparagi

Makes 4 servings

For a more substantial dish, I sometimes top each bundle with slices of Fontina Valle d'Aosta, mozzarella, or another cheese that will melt well.

1 pound asparagus

Salt and freshly ground pepper

4 slices imported Italian prosciutto

2 tablespoons butter

¼ cup freshly grated Parmigiano-Reggiano

1. Trim off the base of the asparagus at the point where the stem turns from white to green. Bring about 2 inches of water to a boil in a large skillet. Add the asparagus and salt to taste. Cook until the asparagus bend slightly when you lift them from the stem end, 4 to 8 minutes. Cooking time will depend on the thickness of the asparagus. Remove the asparagus with tongs. Drain on paper towels and pat them dry.

2. Place a rack in the center of the oven. Preheat the oven to 350°F. Butter a large baking dish.

3. Melt the butter in a large skillet. Add the asparagus and sprinkle them with salt and pepper. Using two spatulas, turn the asparagus carefully in the butter to coat them well.

4. Divide the asparagus into 4 groups. Place each group in the center of a slice of prosciutto. Wrap the ends of the prosciutto around the asparagus. Place the bundles in the baking dish. Sprinkle with the Parmigiano.

5. Bake the asparagus 15 minutes or until the cheese is melted and forms a crust. Serve hot.

Roasted Asparagus

Asparagi al Forno

Makes 4 to 6 servings

Roasting browns the asparagus and brings out their natural sweetness. These are perfect when you are roasting meat. You can remove the cooked meat from the oven, and while it rests, bake the asparagus. Use thick asparagus for this recipe.

1 pound asparagus

¼ cup olive oil

Salt

1. Place a rack in the center of the oven. Preheat the oven to 450°F. Trim off the base of the asparagus at the point where the stem turns from white to green.

2. Place the asparagus in a baking pan large enough to hold them in a single layer. Drizzle with oil and salt. Roll the asparagus from side to side to coat them with the oil.

3. Bake 8 to 10 minutes or until the asparagus are just tender.

Asparagus in Zabaglione

Asparagi allo Zabaione

Makes 6 servings

Zabaglione is a fluffy egg custard that is usually served sweetened for dessert. In this case, the eggs are beaten with white wine and no sugar and served over asparagus. This makes an elegant first course for a spring meal. Peeling the asparagus is optional but ensures that the asparagus will be tender from tip to stem.

1½ pounds asparagus

2 large egg yolks

¼ cup dry white wine

Pinch of salt

1 tablespoon unsalted butter

1. Trim off the base of the asparagus at the point where the stem turns from white to green. To peel the asparagus, start below the tip and, using a swivel-blade peeler, strip away the dark green peel down to the stem end.

2. Bring about 2 inches of water to a boil in a large skillet. Add the asparagus and salt to taste. Cook until the asparagus bend slightly when you lift them from the stem end, 4 to 8 minutes. Cooking time will depend on the thickness of the asparagus. Remove the asparagus with tongs. Drain on paper towels and pat them dry.

3. Bring about an inch of water to a simmer in the bottom half of a double boiler or saucepan. Place the egg yolks, wine, and salt in the top of the double boiler, or in a heatproof bowl that fits comfortably over the saucepan without touching the water.

4. Beat the egg mixture until blended, then place the pan or bowl over the simmering water. Beat with a hand-held electric mixer or with a wire whisk until the mixture is pale-colored and holds a soft shape when the beaters are lifted, about 5 minutes. Beat in the butter just until blended.

5. Spoon the warm sauce over the asparagus and serve immediately.

Asparagus with Taleggio and Pine Nuts

Asparagi con Taleggio e Pinoli

Makes 6 to 8 servings

Not far from Peck's, the famous gastronomia (gourmet food store) in Milan, is the Trattoria Milanese. It is a great place to try simple, classic Lombardian dishes, such as these asparagus topped with taleggio—a buttery, semisoft and aromatic cow's milk cheese that is made locally and is one of Italy's finest cheeses. Fontina or Bel Paese can be substituted if taleggio is not available.

2 pounds asparagus

Salt

2 tablespoons unsalted butter, melted

6 ounces taleggio, Fontina Valle d'Aosta or Bel Paese, cut into bite-size pieces

¼ cup chopped pine nuts or sliced almonds

1 tablespoon plain bread crumbs

1. Place a rack in the center of the oven. Preheat the oven to 450°F. Butter a 13 × 9 × 2–inch baking dish.

2. Trim off the base of the asparagus at the point where the stem turns from white to green. To peel the asparagus, start below the tip and, using a swivel-blade peeler, strip away the dark green peel down to the stem end.

3. Bring about 2 inches of water to a boil in a large skillet. Add the asparagus and salt to taste. Cook until the asparagus bend slightly when you lift them by the stem end, 4 to 8 minutes. Cooking time will depend on the thickness of the asparagus. Remove the asparagus with tongs. Drain them on paper towels and pat them dry.

4. Arrange the asparagus in the baking dish. Drizzle with the butter. Scatter the cheese over the asparagus. Sprinkle with the nuts and bread crumbs.

5. Bake until the cheese is melted and the nuts are browned, about 15 minutes. Serve hot.

Asparagus Timbales

Sformatini di Asparagi

Makes 6 servings

Silky smooth custards like these are an old-fashioned preparation, but one that continues to be popular in many Italian restaurants; essentially because it is very delicious. Practically any vegetable can be made this way, and these little molds are good for a side dish, first course, or vegetarian main dish. Sformatini, literally "little unmolded things," can be served plain, topped with a tomato or cheese sauce, or surrounded with buttery sautéed vegetables.

1 cup Béchamel Sauce

1½ pounds asparagus, trimmed

3 large eggs

¼ cup freshly grated Parmigiano-Reggiano

Salt and freshly ground black pepper

1. Prepare the béchamel, if necessary. Bring about 2 inches of water to a boil in a large skillet. Add the asparagus and salt to taste. Cook until the asparagus bend slightly when you lift them by the stem end, 4 to 8 minutes. Cooking time will depend on the thickness of the asparagus. Remove the asparagus with tongs. Drain them on paper towels and pat them dry. Cut off and set aside 6 of the tips.

2. Place the asparagus in a food processor and process until smooth. Blend in the eggs, béchamel, cheese, 1 teaspoon salt, and pepper to taste.

3. Place a rack in the center of the oven. Preheat the oven to 350°F. Generously butter six 6-ounce ramekins or custard cups. Pour the asparagus mixture into the cups. Place the cups in a large roasting pan and pour boiling water into the pan to reach halfway up the sides of the cups.

4. Bake 50 to 60 minutes or until a knife inserted in the center comes out clean. Remove the molds from the pan and run a small knife around the edge. Invert the molds onto serving dishes. Top with the reserved asparagus tips and serve hot.

Country-Style Beans

Fagioli alla Paesana

Makes about 6 cups of beans, serving 10 to 12

This is a basic cooking method for all types of beans. The soaking beans can ferment if left at room temperature, so I place them in the refrigerator. Once they are cooked, serve them as is with a drizzle of extra-virgin olive oil, or add them to soups or salads.

1 pound cranberry, cannellini, or other dried beans

1 carrot, trimmed

1 celery rib with leaves

1 onion

2 garlic cloves

2 tablespoons olive oil

Salt

1. Rinse the beans and pick them over to remove any broken beans or small stones.

2. Place the beans in a large bowl with cold water to cover by 2 inches. Refrigerate 4 hours up to overnight.

3. Drain the beans and place them in a large pot with fresh cold water to cover by 1 inch. Bring the water to a simmer over medium heat. Reduce the heat to low and skim off the foam that rises to the surface. When the foam stops rising, add the vegetables and olive oil.

4. Cover the pot and simmer $1^1/_2$ to 2 hours, adding more water if needed, until the beans are very tender and creamy. Add salt to taste and let stand about 10 minutes. Discard the vegetables. Serve hot or at room temperature.

Tuscan Beans

Fagioli Stufati

Makes 6 servings

Tuscans are the masters of bean cookery. They slowly simmer the dried legumes with herbs in barely bubbling liquid. Long, slow cooking yields tender, creamy beans that keep their shape as they cook.

Always test several beans to determine doneness, because not all of them will be cooked at the same moment. I let the beans sit awhile on the turned-off stove after cooking to be sure that they are done evenly. They are good when lukewarm, and they reheat perfectly.

Beans are good as a side dish or in soups, or try them spooned over warm toasted Italian bread that has been rubbed with garlic and drizzled with oil.

8 ounces dried cannellini, cranberry, or other beans

1 large garlic clove, slightly crushed

6 fresh sage leaves, or a small branch of rosemary, or 3 sprigs of fresh thyme

Salt

Extra-virgin olive oil

Freshly ground black pepper

1. Rinse the beans and pick them over to remove any broken beans or small stones. Place the beans in a large bowl with cold water to cover by 2 inches. Refrigerate 4 hours up to overnight.

2. Preheat the oven to 300°F. Drain the beans and place them in a Dutch oven or other deep, heavy pot with a tight-fitting lid. Add fresh water to cover by 1 inch. Add the garlic and sage. Bring to a simmer over low heat.

3. Cover the pot and place it on the center rack of the oven. Cook until the beans are very tender, about 1 hour and 15 minutes or more, depending on the type and age of the beans. Check occasionally to see if more water is needed to keep the beans covered. Some beans may require 30 minutes more cooking time.

4. Taste the beans. When they are completely tender, add salt to taste. Let the beans stand for 10 minutes. Serve warm with a drizzle of olive oil and a sprinkle of black pepper.

Bean Salad

Insalata di Fagioli

Makes 4 servings

Dressing the beans while they are warm helps them to absorb the flavors.

2 tablespoons extra-virgin olive oil

2 tablespoons fresh lemon juice

Salt and freshly ground black pepper

2 cups warm cooked or canned beans, such as cannellini or cranberry beans

1 small yellow bell pepper, diced

1 cup cherry tomatoes, halved or quartered

2 green onions, cut into ½-inch pieces

1 bunch arugula, trimmed

1. In a medium bowl, whisk together the oil, lemon juice, and salt and pepper to taste. Drain the beans and add them to the dressing. Stir well. Let stand 30 minutes.

2. Add the pepper, tomatoes, and onions and toss together. Taste and adjust seasoning.

3. Arrange the arugula on a platter and top with the salad. Serve immediately.

Beans and Cabbage

Fagioli e Cavolo

Makes 6 servings

Serve this as a first course in place of pasta or soup, or as a side dish with roast pork or chicken.

2 ounces pancetta (4 thick slices), cut into ½-inch strips

2 tablespoons olive oil

1 small onion, chopped

2 large garlic cloves

¼ teaspoon crushed red pepper

4 cups shredded cabbage

1 cup chopped fresh or canned tomatoes

Salt

3 cups drained cooked or canned cannellini or cranberry beans

1. In a large skillet, cook the pancetta in the olive oil for 5 minutes. Stir in the onion, garlic, and hot pepper and cook until the onion is softened, about 10 minutes.

2. Add the cabbage, tomatoes, and salt to taste. Reduce the heat to low and cover the pan. Cook 20 minutes or until the cabbage is tender. Stir in the beans and cook 5 minutes more. Serve hot.

Beans in Tomato-Sage Sauce

Fagioli all'Uccelletto

Makes 8 servings

These Tuscan beans are cooked in the manner of little game birds, with sage and tomato, hence their Italian name.

1 pound dried cannellini or Great Northern beans, rinsed and picked over

Salt

2 sprigs fresh sage

3 large garlic cloves

¼ cup olive oil

3 large tomatoes, peeled, seeded, and chopped, or 2 cups canned tomatoes

1. Place the beans in a large bowl with cold water to cover by 2 inches. Place them in the refrigerator to soak 4 hours up to overnight.

2. Drain the beans and place them in a large pot with cold water to cover by 1 inch. Bring the liquid to a simmer. Cover and cook until the beans are tender, $1^{1}/_{2}$ to 2 hours. Add salt to taste and let stand 10 minutes.

3. In a large saucepan, cook the sage and garlic in the oil over medium heat, flattening the garlic with the back of a spoon, until the garlic is golden, about 5 minutes. Stir in the tomatoes.

4. Drain the beans, reserving the liquid. Add the beans to the sauce. Cook 10 minutes, adding some of the reserved liquid if the beans become dry. Serve warm or at room temperature.

Chickpea Stew

Ceci in Zimino

Makes 4 to 6 servings

This hearty stew is good on its own, or you can add some cooked small pasta or rice and water or broth to turn it into a soup.

1 medium onion, chopped

1 garlic clove, finely chopped

4 tablespoons olive oil

1 pound Swiss chard or spinach, trimmed and chopped

Salt and freshly ground black pepper

3½ cups drained cooked or canned chickpeas

Extra-virgin olive oil

1. In a medium saucepan, cook the onion and garlic in the oil over medium heat until golden, 10 minutes. Add the Swiss chard and salt to taste. Cover and cook 15 minutes.

2. Add the chickpeas with some of their cooking liquid or water and salt and pepper to taste. Cover and cook 30 minutes more. Stir occasionally and mash some of the chickpeas with the back of a spoon. Add a little more liquid if the mixture becomes too dry.

3. Let cool slightly before serving. Drizzle with a little extra-virgin olive oil if desired

Fava Beans with Bitter Greens

Fave e Cicoria

Makes 4 to 6 servings

Dried fava beans have an earthy, slightly bitter flavor. When buying them, look for the peeled variety. They are slightly more expensive, but are worth it to avoid the tough skins. They also cook more quickly than skin-on favas. You can find dried peeled fava beans in ethnic markets and those specializing in natural foods.

This recipe is from Puglia, where it is practically the national dish. Any kind of bitter greens can be used, such as chicory, broccoli rabe, turnip greens, or dandelion. I like to add a pinch of crushed red pepper to the vegetables as they cook, but that is not traditional.

8 ounces peeled dried fava beans, rinsed and drained

1 medium boiling potato, peeled and cut into 1-inch pieces

Salt

1 pound chicory or dandelion greens, trimmed

¼ cup extra-virgin olive oil

1 garlic clove, finely chopped

Pinch of crushed red pepper

1. Place the beans and potato in a large pot. Add cold water to cover by $1/2$ inch. Bring to a simmer and cook until the beans are very soft and falling apart and all the water is absorbed.

2. Add salt to taste. Mash the beans with the back of a spoon or a potato masher. Stir in the oil.

3. Bring a large pot of water to a boil. Add the greens and salt to taste. Cook until tender, depending on the variety of greens, 5 to 10 minutes. Drain well.

4. Dry the pot. Add the oil, garlic, and crushed red pepper. Cook over medium heat until the garlic is golden, about 2 minutes. Add the drained greens and salt to taste. Toss well.

5. Spread the bean puree on a serving platter. Pile the greens on top. Drizzle with more oil if desired. Serve hot or warm.

Fresh Fava Beans, Roman Style

Fave alla Romana

Makes 4 servings

Fresh fava beans in their pods are an important spring vegetable throughout central and southern Italy. The Romans like to pop them out of the shells and eat them raw as an accompaniment to young pecorino cheese. The beans are also stewed with other spring vegetables such as peas and artichokes.

If the fava beans are very young and tender, it is not necessary to peel off the thin skin that covers each bean. Try eating one with the peel and another without it to decide if they are tender.

The flavor and texture of fresh favas is completely different from dried favas, so do not substitute one for the other. If you can't find fresh favas, look for the frozen beans sold in many Italian and Middle Eastern markets. Fresh or frozen lima beans also work well in this dish.

1 small onion, finely chopped

4 ounces pancetta, diced

2 tablespoons olive oil

4 pounds fresh fava beans, shelled (about 3 cups)

Salt and freshly ground black pepper

¼ cup water

1. In a medium skillet, cook the onion and pancetta in the olive oil over medium heat for 10 minutes or until golden.

2. Stir in the fava beans and salt and pepper to taste. Add the water and lower the heat. Cover the pan and cook 5 minutes or until the beans are almost tender.

3. Uncover the pan and cook until the beans and pancetta are lightly browned, about 5 minutes. Serve hot.

Fresh Fava Beans, Umbrian Style

Scafata

Makes 6 servings

Fava bean pods should be firm and crisp, not wrinkled or soft, which indicates that they are too old. The smaller the pod, the more tender the beans. Figure Bout 1 pound of fresh favas in the pod for 1 cup shelled favas.

2½ pounds fresh fava beans, shelled, or 2 cups frozen favas

1 pound Swiss chard, trimmed and cut in ½-inch strips

1 onion, chopped

1 medium carrot, chopped

1 celery rib, chopped

¼ cup olive oil

1 teaspoon salt

Freshly ground black pepper

1 medium ripe tomato, peeled, seeded, and chopped

1. In a medium saucepan, stir together all of the ingredients except the tomato. Cover and cook over low heat, stirring occasionally, for 15 minutes or until the beans are tender. Add a little water if the vegetables begin to stick.

2. Stir in the tomato and cook uncovered for 5 minutes. Serve hot.

Broccoli with Oil and Lemon

Broccoli al Agro

Makes 6 servings

This is the basic way of serving many types of cooked green vegetables in southern Italy. They are always served at room temperature.

1½ pounds broccoli

Salt

¼ cup extra-virgin olive oil

1 to 2 tablespoons fresh lemon juice

Lemon wedges, for garnish

1. Cut the broccoli into large florets. Trim off the ends of the stems. Peel off the tough skin with a swivel-blade vegetable peeler. Cut thick stems crosswise into $1/4$-inch slices.

2. Bring a large pot of water to a boil. Add the broccoli and salt to taste. Cook until the broccoli is tender, 5 to 7 minutes. Drain and cool slightly under cold running water.

3. Drizzle the broccoli with the oil and lemon juice. Garnish with the lemon wedges. Serve at room temperature.

Broccoli, Parma Style

Broccoli alla Parmigiana

Makes 4 servings

For variety, make this dish with a combination of cauliflower and broccoli.

1½ pounds broccoli

Salt

3 tablespoons unsalted butter

Freshly ground black pepper

½ cup freshly grated Parmigiano-Reggiano

1. Cut the broccoli into large florets. Trim off the ends of the stems. Peel off the tough skin with a swivel-blade vegetable peeler. Cut thick stems crosswise into $1/4$-inch slices.

2. Bring a large pot of water to a boil. Add the broccoli and salt to taste. Cook until the broccoli is partially done, about 5 minutes. Drain and cool under cold water.

3. Place a rack in the center of the oven. Preheat the oven to 375°F. Butter a baking dish large enough to hold the broccoli.

4. Arrange the spears in the prepared dish, overlapping them slightly. Dot with the butter and sprinkle with pepper. Sprinkle the cheese on top.

5. Bake 10 minutes or until the cheese is melted and slightly browned. Serve hot.

Broccoli Rabe with Garlic and Hot Pepper

Cime di Rape col Peperoncino

Makes 4 servings

It doesn't get much better than this recipe when it comes to seasoning broccoli rabe. This dish can also be made with regular broccoli or cauliflower. Some versions include a few anchovies sautéed with the garlic and oil, or try adding a handful of olives for a salty tang. This also makes a great topping for pasta.

1½ pounds broccoli rabe

Salt

3 tablespoons olive oil

2 large garlic cloves, thinly sliced

Pinch of crushed red pepper

1. Separate the broccoli rabe into florets. Trim off the base of the stems. Peeling the stems is optional. Cut each floret crosswise into 2 or 3 pieces.

2. Bring a large pot of water to a boil. Add the broccoli rabe and salt to taste. Cook until the broccoli is almost tender, about 5 minutes. Drain.

3. Dry the pot and add the oil, garlic, and red pepper. Cook over medium heat until the garlic is lightly golden, about 2 minutes. Add the broccoli and a sprinkle of salt. Stir well. Cover and cook until tender, 3 minutes more. Serve hot or at room temperature.

Broccoli with Prosciutto

Brasato di Broccoli

Makes 4 servings

The broccoli in this recipe is cooked until it is soft enough to mash with a fork. Serve it as a side dish or spread it on toasted Italian bread for crostini.

1½ pounds broccoli

Salt

¼ cup olive oil

1 medium onion, chopped

1 garlic clove, finely chopped

4 thin slices imported Italian prosciutto, cut crosswise into thin strips

1. Cut the broccoli into large florets. Trim off the ends of the stems. Peel off the tough skin with a swivel-blade vegetable peeler. Cut thick stems crosswise into ¼-inch slices.

2. Bring a large pot of water to a boil. Add the broccoli and salt to taste. Cook until the broccoli is partially done, about 5 minutes. Drain and cool under cold water.

3. Dry the pot and add the oil, onion, and garlic. Cook over medium heat until golden, about 10 minutes. Stir in the broccoli. Cover and turn the heat to low. Cook until the broccoli is soft, about 15 minutes.

4. Coarsely mash the broccoli with a potato masher or a fork. Stir in the prosciutto. Season to taste with salt and pepper. Serve hot.

Bread Bites with Broccoli Rabe

Morsi con Cime di Rape

Makes 4 servings

A minestra can be a thick soup made with pasta or rice, or a hearty vegetable dish, such as this one from Puglia containing cubes of bread. Though it was probably invented by a thrifty housewife with leftover bread and many mouths to fill, it is tasty enough for a first course or as a side dish with pork ribs or chops.

1½ pounds broccoli rabe

3 garlic cloves, thinly sliced

Pinch of crushed red pepper

⅓ cup olive oil

4 to 6 (½-inch-thick) slices Italian or French bread, cut into bite-size pieces

1. Separate the broccoli rabe into florets. Trim off the base of the stems. Peeling the stems is optional. Cut each floret crosswise into 1-inch pieces.

2. Bring a large pot of water to a boil. Add the broccoli rabe and salt to taste. Cook until the broccoli is almost tender, about 5 minutes. Drain.

3. In a large skillet, cook the garlic and red pepper in the oil for 1 minute. Stir in the bread cubes and cook, stirring often until the bread is lightly toasted, about 3 minutes.

4. Stir in the broccoli rabe and a pinch of salt. Cook, stirring, 5 minutes more. Serve hot.

Broccoli Rabe with Pancetta and Tomatoes

Cime di Rape al Pomodori

Makes 4 servings

In this recipe, the meaty flavor of pancetta, onion, and tomato complements the bold flavor of the broccoli rabe. This is another one of those dishes that would be great tossed with some hot cooked pasta.

1½ pounds broccoli rabe

Salt

2 tablespoons olive oil

2 thick slices pancetta, chopped

1 medium onion, chopped

Pinch of crushed red pepper

1 cup chopped canned tomatoes

2 tablespoons dry white wine or water

1. Separate the broccoli rabe into florets. Trim off the base of the stems. Peeling the stems is optional. Cut each floret crosswise into 1-inch pieces.

2. Bring a large pot of water to a boil. Add the broccoli rabe and salt to taste. Cook until the broccoli is almost tender, about 5 minutes. Drain.

3. Pour the oil into a large skillet. Add the pancetta, onion, and red pepper and cook over medium heat until the onion is translucent, about 5 minutes. Add the tomatoes, wine, and a pinch of salt. Cook 10 minutes more or until thickened.

4. Stir in the broccoli rabe and cook until heated, about 2 minutes. Serve hot.

Little Vegetable Cakes

Frittelle di Erbe di Campo

Makes 8 servings

In Sicily, these little vegetable pancakes are made with bitter wild greens. You can use broccoli rabe, mustard greens, borage, or chicory. These little cakes are traditionally eaten at Easter time as an appetizer or side dish. They are good hot or at room temperature.

1½ pounds broccoli rabe

Salt

4 large eggs

2 tablespoons grated caciocavallo or Pecorino Romano

Salt and freshly ground black pepper

2 tablespoons olive oil

1. Separate the broccoli rabe into florets. Trim off the base of the stems. Peeling the stems is optional. Cut each floret crosswise into 1-inch pieces.

2. Bring a large pot of water to a boil. Add the broccoli rabe and salt to taste. Cook until the broccoli is almost tender, about 5 minutes. Drain. Let cool slightly, then press out the water. Chop broccoli rabe.

3. In a large bowl, whisk the eggs, cheese, and salt and pepper to taste. Stir in the greens.

4. Heat the oil in a large skillet over medium heat. Scoop up a heaping tablespoonful of the mixture and place it in the pan. Flatten the mixture with a spoon into a small pancake. Repeat with the remaining mixture. Cook 1 side of the cakes until lightly browned, about 2 minutes, then turn them over with a spatula and cook the other side until browned and cooked through. Serve hot or at room temperature.

Fried Cauliflower

Cavolfiore Fritte

Makes 4 servings

Try serving cauliflower prepared this way to someone who does not normally like this versatile vegetable, and you are sure to make a convert. The crisp, cheese-flavored coating provides an excellent contrast to the tender cauliflower. These can be passed as party appetizers or served as a side dish with grilled chops. For best texture, serve them immediately after cooking.

1 small cauliflower (about 1 pound)

Salt

1 cup plain dry bread crumbs

3 large eggs

$\frac{1}{2}$ cup freshly grated Parmigiano-Reggiano

Freshly ground black pepper

Vegetable oil

Lemon wedges

1. Cut the cauliflower into 2-inch florets. Trim off the ends of the stems. Cut thick stems crosswise into $1/4$-inch slices.

2. Bring a large pot of water to a boil. Add the cauliflower and salt to taste. Cook until the cauliflower is almost tender, about 5 minutes. Drain and cool under cold water.

3. Put the bread crumbs in a shallow plate. In a small bowl, whisk the eggs, cheese, and salt and pepper to taste. Dip the cauliflower pieces in the egg, then roll them in the bread crumbs. Let dry on a rack for 15 minutes.

4. Pour the oil into a large deep skillet to a depth of $1/2$ inch. Heat over medium heat until a bit of the egg mixture dropped into the pan sizzles and cooks rapidly. Meanwhile, line a tray with paper towels.

5. Place only enough pieces of cauliflower in the pan as will fit comfortably without touching. Fry the pieces, turning them with tongs, until golden brown and crisp all over, about 6 minutes. Drain the cauliflower on the paper towels. Repeat with the remaining cauliflower.

6. Serve the cauliflower hot, with lemon wedges.

Cauliflower Puree

Purèa di Cavolfiore

Makes 4 servings

Though it looks like ordinary mashed potatoes, this puree of cauliflower and potatoes is much lighter and more flavorful. It is a nice change from mashed potatoes and could even be served with a hearty stew, such as Braised Beef Shank.

1 small cauliflower (about 1 pound)

3 medium boiling potatoes, peeled and quartered

Salt

1 tablespoon unsalted butter

2 tablespoons grated Parmigiano-Reggiano

Freshly ground black pepper

1. Cut the cauliflower into 2-inch florets. Trim off the ends of the stems. Cut thick stems crosswise into $1/4$-inch slices.

2. In a pot large enough to hold all the vegetables, combine the potatoes with 3 quarts cold water and salt to taste. Bring to a simmer and cook 5 minutes.

3. Add the cauliflower and cook until the vegetables are very tender, about 10 minutes. Drain the cauliflower and potatoes. Blend them until smooth with an electric mixer or hand-held blender. Do not overbeat them or the potatoes will become gluey.

4. Stir in the butter, cheese, and salt and pepper to taste. Serve hot.

Roasted Cauliflower

Cavolfiore al Forno

Makes 4 to 6 servings

Cauliflower goes from bland to delicious when it is roasted until lightly browned. For variation, toss the cooked cauliflower with a little balsamic vinegar.

1 medium cauliflower (about 1½ pounds)

¼ cup olive oil

Salt and freshly ground black pepper

1. Cut the cauliflower into 2-inch florets. Trim off the ends of the stems. Cut thick stems crosswise into $1/4$-inch slices.

2. Place a rack in the center of the oven. Preheat the oven to 350°F. Spread the cauliflower in a roasting pan just large enough to hold it in single layer. Toss with the oil and a generous sprinkle of salt and pepper.

3. Bake, stirring occasionally, for 45 minutes or until the cauliflower is tender and lightly browned. Serve warm.

Smothered Cauliflower

Cavolfiore Stufato

Makes 4 to 6 servings

Some people say that cauliflower is bland, but I say that its mild flavor and creamy texture is a perfect backdrop for flavorful ingredients.

1 medium cauliflower (about 1½ pounds)

3 tablespoons olive oil

¼ cup water

2 garlic cloves, thinly sliced

Salt

½ cup mild black olives, such as Gaeta, pitted and sliced

4 anchovies, chopped (optional)

2 tablespoons chopped fresh flat-leaf parsley

1. Cut the cauliflower into 2-inch florets. Trim off the ends of the stems. Cut thick stems crosswise into ¹/₄-inch slices.

2. Pour the oil into a large skillet and add the cauliflower. Cook over medium heat until the cauliflower begins to brown. Add the water, garlic, and a pinch of salt. Cover and cook over low heat until the cauliflower is tender when pierced with a knife and the water has evaporated, about 10 minutes.

3. Add the olives, anchovies, and parsley and toss well. Cook uncovered 2 minutes more, stirring occasionally. Serve hot.

Cauliflower with Parsley and Onion

Cavolfiore Trifolato

Makes 4 to 6 servings

The onion, garlic, and parsley infuse this cauliflower with flavor as they all steam together gently in the pan.

1 medium cauliflower (about 1½ pounds)

2 tablespoons olive oil

1 medium onion, thinly sliced

2 garlic cloves, finely chopped

2 tablespoons water

¼ cup chopped fresh flat-leaf parsley

Salt and freshly ground black pepper

1. Cut the cauliflower into 2-inch florets. Trim off the ends of the stems. Peel off the tough skin with a swivel-blade vegetable peeler. Cut thick stems crosswise into 1/4-inch slices.

2. In a large skillet, cook the onion and garlic in the olive oil and cook 5 minutes, stirring occasionally.

3. Add the cauliflower, water, parsley, and salt and pepper to taste. Toss well. Cover the pan and cook 15 minutes more or until the cauliflower is tender. Serve hot.

Cauliflower in Tomato Sauce

Cavolfiore in Salsa

Makes 6 to 8 servings

If you like, add a handful of drained capers to the sauce for this dish. It is also good served as a pasta sauce, topped with a sprinkle of toasted bread crumbs.

1 medium cauliflower (about 1½ pounds)

1 medium onion, chopped

2 garlic cloves, finely chopped

Pinch of crushed red pepper

2 tablespoons olive oil

1 (28-ounce) can peeled tomatoes, chopped

Salt

2 tablespoons chopped fresh basil or flat-leaf parsley

1. Cut the cauliflower into 2-inch florets. Trim off the ends of the stems. Cut thick stems crosswise into ¹/₄-inch slices.

2. In a large saucepan, cook the onion, garlic, and crushed red pepper in the oil over medium heat, stirring occasionally, until the onion is tender, about 10 minutes. Stir in the tomatoes. Bring to a simmer. Cook 10 minutes.

3. Stir in the cauliflower and basil or parsley, and salt to taste. Cover and cook 15 minutes, stirring occasionally. Uncover and cook 5 minutes more.

Cauliflower Torte

Tortino di Cavolfiore

Makes 6 servings

Enormous, creamy white heads of cauliflower are piled high at my local farmer's market each fall. They remind me to make this excellent dish, which I first had in Tuscany. When baked, it looks like a golden cake and cuts neatly into squares.

1 large cauliflower (about 2 pounds)

Salt

¼ cup olive oil

2 large garlic cloves, finely chopped

3 tablespoons plain dry bread crumbs

4 large eggs

½ cup freshly grated Parmigiano-Reggiano

Freshly ground black pepper

1. Cut the cauliflower into 2-inch florets. Trim off the ends of the stems. Cut thick stems crosswise into $1/4$-inch slices.

2. Bring a large pot of water to a boil. Add the cauliflower and salt to taste. Cook until the cauliflower is soft, about 15 minutes. Drain well. Place the cauliflower in a large bowl and mash it with a potato masher or the back of a spoon. It should not be perfectly smooth.

3. Pour the oil into a small skillet. Add the garlic and cook over medium heat until golden, about 2 minutes. Scrape the garlic and oil into the cauliflower and stir well.

4. Place a rack in the center of the oven. Preheat the oven to 400°F. Oil a 9-inch square baking pan. Sprinkle the pan with one tablespoon of the crumbs. Beat together the eggs, cheese, and salt and pepper to taste. Stir the egg mixture into the cauliflower. Scrape the mixture into the pan and smooth the top. Sprinkle with the remaining crumbs.

5. Bake 30 to 35 minutes or until a knife inserted in the center comes out clean and the top is lightly browned. Let cool 10 minutes. Cut into squares and serve hot or at room temperature.

Brussels Sprouts with Butter

Cavolini di Bruxelles al Burro

Makes 4 to 6 servings

When boiling brussels sprouts, it is important not to overcook them, as their flavor and odor will become overpowering. Add lemon juice, herbs, garlic, or mustard to the butter if you like. You can also sprinkle the buttered sprouts with Parmigiano-Reggiano and leave them covered for a minute until the cheese melts.

1 pound brussels sprouts

Salt

2 tablespoons unsalted butter

Freshly ground black pepper

1. With a small knife, shave a thin slice off the base of the brussels sprouts. Cut them in half through the base.

2. Bring a large pot of water to a boil. Add the brussels sprouts and salt to taste. Cook until the sprouts are tender when pierced with a knife, 6 to 8 minutes.

3. Melt the butter in a large skillet over medium heat. Add the sprouts and salt and pepper to taste. Cook 2 to 3 minutes, shaking the pan occasionally. Serve hot.

PASTRIES AND DESSERTS

Poached Pears with Gorgonzola

Pere al Gorgonzola

Makes 4 servings

The spicy flavor of gorgonzola cheese blended to a smooth cream is a savory complement to these pears poached in a lemony white-wine syrup. A sprinkling of pistachios adds a bright touch of color. Anjou, Bartlett, and Bosc pears are my favorite varieties for poaching, because their slender shape allows them to cook through evenly. Poached pears hold their shape better when the fruit are not too ripe.

2 cups dry white wine

2 tablespoons fresh lemon juice

¾ cup sugar

2 (2-inch) strips lemon zest

4 pears, such as Anjou, Bartlett, or Bosc

4 ounces gorgonzola

2 tablespoons ricotta, mascarpone, or heavy cream

2 tablespoons chopped pistachios

1. In a medium saucepan, combine the wine, lemon juice, sugar, and lemon zest. Bring to a simmer and cook for 10 minutes.

2. Meanwhile, peel the pears and cut them in half lengthwise. Remove the cores.

3. Slip the pears into the wine syrup and cook until tender when pierced with a knife, about 10 minutes. Let cool.

4. With a slotted spoon, transfer two pear halves to each serving dish, cored-side up. Drizzle the syrup around the pears.

5. In a small bowl, mash the gorgonzola with the ricotta to make a smooth paste. Scoop some of the cheese mixture into the cored space of each pear half. Sprinkle with the pistachios. Serve immediately.

Pear or Apple Pudding Cake

Budino di Pere o Mele

Makes 6 servings

Not quite a cake or a pudding, this dessert consists of fruit cooked until tender, then baked with a slightly cakelike topping. It is good with apples or pears or even peaches or plums.

I like to use dark rum for flavoring this dessert, but light rum, cognac, or even grappa can be substituted.

¾ cup raisins

½ cup dark rum, cognac, or grappa

2 tablespoons unsalted butter

8 firm ripe pears or apples, peeled and cut into ½-inch slices

⅓ cup sugar

Topping

6 tablespoons unsalted butter, melted and cooled

⅓ cup sugar

½ cup all-purpose flour

3 large eggs, separated

⅔ cup whole milk

2 tablespoons dark rum, cognac, or grappa

1 teaspoon pure vanilla extract

Pinch of salt

Confectioner's sugar

1. In a small bowl, toss together the raisins and rum. Let stand for 30 minutes.

2. Melt the butter in a large skillet over medium heat. Add the fruit and sugar. Cook, stirring occasionally, until the fruit is almost tender, about 7 minutes. Add the raisins and rum. Cook 2 minutes more. Remove from the heat.

3. Place a rack in the center of the oven. Preheat the oven to 350°F. Grease a 13 × 9 × 2–inch baking dish. Spoon the fruit mixture into the baking dish.

4. Prepare the topping: In a large bowl, with an electric mixer, beat the butter and sugar until blended, about 3 minutes. Stir in the flour, just to combine.

5. In a medium bowl, whisk together the egg yolks, milk, rum, and vanilla. Stir the egg mixture into the flour mixture until blended.

6. In another large bowl, with clean beaters beat the egg whites with the salt on low speed until foamy. Increase the speed and beat until soft peaks form, about 4 minutes. Gently fold the whites into the rest of the batter. Pour the batter over the fruit in the baking dish and bake 25 minutes or until the top is golden and firm to the touch.

7. Serve warm or at room temperature, sprinkled with confectioner's sugar.

Warm Fruit Compote

Composta di Frutta Calda

Makes 6 to 8 servings

Rum is often used to flavor desserts in Italy. Dark rum has a deeper flavor than light rum. Substitute another liqueur or a sweet wine such as Marsala for the rum in this recipe if you like. Or make a nonalcoholic version with orange or apple juice.

2 firm ripe pears, peeled and cored

1 golden delicious or Granny Smith apple, peeled and cored

1 cup pitted prunes

1 cup dried figs, stem ends removed

½ cup dried pitted apricots

½ cup dark raisins

¼ cup sugar

2 (2-inch) strips lemon zest

1 cup water

½ cup dark rum

1. Cut the pears and apple into 8 wedges. Cut the wedges into bite-size pieces.

2. Combine all of the ingredients in a large saucepan. Cover and bring to a simmer over medium-low heat. Cook until the fresh fruits are tender and the dried fruits are plump, about 20 minutes. Add a little more water if they seem dry.

3. Let cool slightly before serving or cover and refrigerate up to 3 days.

Venetian Caramelized Fruit

Golosezzi Veneziani

Makes 8 servings

The caramel coating on these Venetian skewered fruits hardens, with a result something like a candy apple. Pat the fruits thoroughly dry and make these fruit skewers on a dry day. If the weather is humid, the caramel will not harden properly.

1 tangerine or clementine, peeled, divided into sections

8 small strawberries, hulled

8 seedless grapes

8 pitted dates

1 cup sugar

½ cup light corn syrup

¼ cup water

1. Thread the fruit pieces alternately on each of eight 6-inch wood skewers. Set a wire cooling rack on top of a tray.

2. In a skillet large enough to fit the skewers into lengthwise, combine the sugar, corn syrup, and water. Cook over medium heat, stirring occasionally until the sugar is completely dissolved, about 3 minutes. When the mixture begins to boil, stop stirring and cook until the syrup starts to brown around the edges. Then gently swirl the pan over the heat until the syrup is an even golden brown, about 2 minutes more.

3. Remove the pan from the heat. Using tongs, quickly dip each skewer in the syrup, turning to coat the fruit lightly but thoroughly. Let the excess syrup drain back into the pan. Place the skewers on the rack to cool. (If the syrup in the pan hardens before all of the skewers have been dipped, reheat it gently.) Serve at room temperature within 2 hours.

Fruit with Honey and Grappa

Composta di Frutta alla Grappa

Makes 6 servings

Grappa is a kind of brandy made from vinaccia, the skins and seeds that are left after grapes are pressed to make wine. At one time, grappa was a coarse beverage mostly drunk in northern Italy by farmhands and laborers for warmth on cold winter days. Today, grappa is a very refined drink, sold in designer bottles with ornate stoppers. Some grappas are flavored with fruit or herbs, while others are aged in wood casks. Use a simple, unflavored grappa for this fruit salad and for other cooking purposes.

⅓ cup honey

⅓ cup grappa, brandy, or fruit liqueur

1 tablespoon fresh lemon juice

2 kiwis, peeled and sliced

2 navel oranges, peeled and cut into wedges

1 pint strawberries, sliced

1 cup halved seedless green grapes

2 medium bananas, sliced

1. In a large serving bowl, mix together the honey, grappa, and
lemon juice.

2. Stir in the kiwis, oranges, strawberries, and grapes. Chill for at
least 1 hour or up to 4 hours. Stir in the bananas just before
serving.

Winter Fruit Salad

Macedonia del' Inverno

Makes 6 servings

In Italy, a fruit salad is called Macedonia, because that country was once divided up into many little sections that were brought together to make a whole, just as the salad is made up of bite-size pieces of different fruits. In the winter, when fruit choices are limited, Italians make salads like this one dressed with honey and lemon juice. As a variation, substitute apricot jam or orange marmalade for the honey.

3 tablespoons honey

3 tablespoons orange juice

1 tablespoon fresh lemon juice

2 grapefruits, peeled and separated into wedges

2 kiwis, peeled and sliced

2 ripe pears

2 cups seedless green grapes, halved lengthwise

1. In a large bowl, mix together the honey, orange juice, and lemon juice.

2. Add the fruits to the bowl and toss well. Chill for at least 1 hour or up to 4 hours before serving.

Grilled Summer Fruit

Spiedini alla Frutta

Makes 6 servings

Grilled summer fruits are great for a barbecue. Serve them plain or with slices of sponge cake and ice cream.

If using wood skewers, soak them in cold water at least 30 minutes to prevent burning.

2 nectarines, cut into 1-inch chunks

2 plums, cut into 1-inch chunks

2 pears, cut into 1-inch chunks

2 apricots, cut into quarters

2 bananas, cut into 1-inch chunks

Fresh mint leaves

About 2 tablespoons sugar

1. Place a barbecue grill or broiler rack about 5 inches away from the heat source. Preheat the grill or broiler.

2. Alternate pieces of the fruits with the mint leaves on 6 skewers. Sprinkle with the sugar.

3. Grill or broil the fruit 3 minutes on one side. Turn the skewers and grill or broil until lightly browned, about 2 minutes more. Serve hot.

Warm Ricotta with Honey

Ricotta al Miele

Makes 2 to 3 servings

The success of this dessert depends on the quality of the ricotta, so buy the freshest available. While part-skimmed-milk ricotta is fine, the fat-free is very grainy and tasteless, so don't use it. If you like, add some fresh fruit, or try raisins and a pinch of cinnamon.

1 cup whole-milk ricotta

2 tablespoons honey

1. Place the ricotta in a small bowl set over a smaller pan of simmering water. Heat until warm, about 10 minutes. Stir well.

2. Scoop the ricotta into serving dishes. Drizzle with the honey. Serve immediately.

Coffee Ricotta

Ricotta all' Caffè

Makes 2 to 3 servings

Here is a quick dessert that lends itself to a multitude of variations. Serve it with some plain butter cookies.

If you can't buy finely ground espresso, be sure to run the grounds through your coffee grinder or food processor. If the grounds are too large, the dessert won't blend right, leaving it with a gritty texture.

1 cup (8 ounces) whole or part-skim ricotta

1 tablespoon finely ground (espresso) coffee

1 tablespoon sugar

Chocolate shavings

In a medium bowl, whisk together the ricotta, espresso, and sugar until the mixture is smooth and the sugar is dissolved. (For a creamier texture, mix the ingredients in a food processor.) Spoon into parfait glasses or goblets and top with chocolate shavings. Serve immediately.

Variation: For chocolate ricotta, substitute 1 tablespoon unsweetened cocoa for the coffee.

Mascarpone and Peaches

Mascarpone al Pesche

Makes 6 servings

Smooth, creamy mascarpone and peaches with crunchy amaretti look beautiful in parfait or wine glasses. Serve this dessert at a dinner party. No one will guess how easy it is to make.

1 cup (8 ounces) mascarpone

$\frac{1}{4}$ cup sugar

1 tablespoon fresh lemon juice

1 cup very cold whipping cream

3 peaches or nectarines, peeled and cut into bite-size pieces

$\frac{1}{3}$ cup orange liqueur, amaretto, or rum

8 amaretti cookies, crushed into crumbs (about $\frac{1}{2}$ cup)

2 tablespoons toasted sliced almonds

1. At least 20 minutes before you are ready to make the dessert, place a large bowl and the beaters of an electric mixer in the refrigerator.

2. When ready, in a medium bowl, whisk together the mascarpone, sugar, and lemon juice. Remove the bowl and beaters from the refrigerator. Pour the cream into the chilled bowl and whip the cream at high speed until it holds its shape softly when the beaters are lifted, about 4 minutes. With a spatula, gently fold the whipped cream into the mascarpone mixture.

3. In a medium bowl, toss together the peaches and liqueur.

4. Spoon half of the mascarpone cream into six parfait glasses or wine goblets. Make a layer of the peaches, then sprinkle with the amaretti crumbs. Top with the remaining cream. Cover and chill in the refrigerator up to 2 hours.

5. Sprinkle with the almonds before serving.